The Key

To

Permanent Slimness

Visit: www.permanentslimness.com

By

Peter Kitson

Published

By

Pageturner Publications

27 Old Gloucester Street, London WC1 3XX

www.pageturnerpublications.com

ISBN- 0-9552967-0-6

Copyright © 2006 Peter Kitson

All rights reserved

1

Prepare Yourself For A Shock:

Probably everything you have ever read or heard on the subject of getting and staying slim has been completely, utterly, and totally wrong.

You have probably suffered (as I did for 30 years) trying to stick to the latest diet or exercise regime, all of which ultimately failed, leaving you disappointed, unhappy, and just as heavy as you were when you started.

You will know only too well the pain of looking in the mirror and feeling unhappy with the shape of your body, and the frustration of not being able to do anything about it. Perhaps you feel guilty or dislike yourself for not having

The Key To Permanent Slimness

the willpower to become and stay slim.

Well I have some good news for you: You can stop beating yourself up – you are not to blame for this!

You have been fed a stream of wrong information and bad advice that, rather than help you get slim, has actually contrived in keeping you fat.

You will not find amongst these pages countless recipes for low-calorie or low-carbohydrate meals, exercise plans, food supplements, or any of the useless paraphernalia we are peddled to lose weight. You don't need any of it. Soon you will be able to free up some shelf space and dump your diet books for all time. You will see how damaging they have been to your attempts to shed those unwanted pounds.

But if you are to reap the same life-changing benefits that I have from the key to permanent slimness, you will need to understand it fully, and more importantly, EXPERIENCE it. The purpose of this book is to

The Key To Permanent Slimness

make that happen. I promise you that a profound and lasting change is about to be made to your weight, your body shape, and your enjoyment of life.

There is a secret to becoming and remaining slim, and it is nothing to do with dieting, exercise, or willpower. The key to permanent slimness is something that might at first seem insignificant, and yet its effect is so powerful that it will catapult you into a slim new world from which there will be no going back. At last you will be free from worries about your weight and will be able to get on with the business of living!

I am going to take you through the thinking process that lead to the discovery of this secret, thereby embedding it permanently in your conscious mind. This is not about losing a few pounds this week, only to put them back on again next week. This is about becoming permanently and naturally slim for the rest of your life.

We are going to apply some rational

thought to the whole problem of obesity, and in the process you will come to understand its true nature.

But before we begin our journey, let's define exactly where we want to go.

2

The World Of The Naturally Slim

Can you imagine being one of the naturally slim? By that I mean one of those people who never seem to put on weight no matter what they eat. Just think for a moment what it would be like to live in their world.

You could go out for meals as often as you liked and pick from the menu what you *want* to eat, not what was low in carbohydrates, low in sugar, or low in anything else. Imagine leaving the table always feeling satisfied, never worrying about what the scales might tell you in the morning.

How about shopping for clothes? You

could buy all the latest fashions knowing they will always hang perfectly on your body and make you look great. No more choosing garments to hide your unwanted bumps.

How would you feel on holiday, stepping out onto the beach wearing your new swimsuit, enjoying the looks of admiration coming your way from people wondering how you manage to keep such a great figure?

How much more confident would you feel in social situations, always looking people in the eye, giving them a warm handshake and a confident smile as they compliment you on your appearance?

At work wouldn't you be more positive and self-assured if you were slim and fit? If you looked like a 'winner' perhaps it would be easier to ask for that raise or promotion.

And then of course there is your love life. Wouldn't you feel more free and liberated when making love to your partner, knowing you didn't have to worry about your thighs looking big, or if your love handles are showing?

The Key To Permanent Slimness

Sounds great doesn't it? Welcome to the world of the naturally slim. The goal of this book is to take you there.

3

The Beginnings Of Discovery

Some years ago I lived with a woman who was naturally slim. She enjoyed her food, was an accomplished cook, and deprived herself of nothing - and yet she never gained weight. Occasionally she would buy herself treats such as a family-sized bar of chocolate, or a sponge cake, oozing with jam and cream. Whenever I opened the fridge (often in the middle of the night) and found myself confronted with such delicacies, I would be left wide-eyed with a mixture of horror and delight – like a heroin addict stumbling across a stash of illicit drugs whilst trying to quit his habit.

Such enticements were always too great for me, and I would devour half the cake or the whole bar of chocolate in five minutes flat.

In the morning we would have the inevitable argument when, racked with guilt, I would express my frustration at the lack of understanding she had shown me by putting temptation in my way. I was on a diet for heaven's sake! She would look at me, open mouthed in disbelief, unable to comprehend why I had felt the need to make such a pig of myself. Bingeing on food really was an alien concept to her.

The difference in the way we related to food puzzled me. Why was she able to take one square of chocolate, enjoy it, and then put the rest of the bar back in the fridge, with no compulsion to finish it off in one go?

It was not a question of willpower – she didn't need any because she never had any cravings to overcome in the first place. This both fascinated and annoyed me. Why were we so different in the way we related to food? Was it just that I was unlucky to be born with an addictive personality, or was I missing something? She sailed through life enjoying her food, free from worries about putting on weight, whilst I put on a couple of pounds whenever I so much as looked at the foods I really enjoyed. Was I destined to a life of feeling either constantly deprived of food, or desperately unhappy with my weight? It seemed so unjust.

Some years later I lived with a girl who had the figure of a fashion model and was also naturally slim. Her answer to the problem of obesity was simple: Eat less and move more.

Oh, if only it were that easy!

When she said this she wasn't trying to be glib – she genuinely had no comprehension of what it is like to have a compulsion to overeat. It was apparent that she had never given any serious thought to the problem of obesity. But then why would she? If you are permanently slim why waste valuable time thinking about a problem that doesn't exist for you?

The Key To Permanent Slimness

I began to realise that the naturally slim have a completely different experience of life to those of us who put on weight, and I tried to imagine what it would be like to be free of the nagging discontentment I had had with my body throughout my adult life.

My imagination kicked in, and for a brief moment I seemed to catch a glimpse of a different, brighter life. Charged with excitement, I became fixated by the idea of a world in which obesity was a thing of the past and slimness was the natural state for EVERY human being. I set out to determine if such a thing were possible, and if so, exactly how it could be achieved.

But there was one question that had to be addressed before all others.

4

Is It All A Question Of Genetics?

Before trying to discover what the key to permanent slimness might be, I had to determine if there actually was a secret to discover in the first place. If it were all down to the lottery of genetics then all of us who were overweight would have to give up the quest for slimness and resign ourselves to our fate. We would be prisoners of our genetic inheritance with no hope whatsoever for change.

It was not a pleasant thought.

When referring to the naturally slim, I had often heard people say that he or she was just "born lucky."

Was this true?

Taking some lessons from the animal kingdom, I applied some logical thinking to this question.

It occurred to me that animals in the wild don't get fat. If they did they would be unable to hunt and would easily be captured by predators. Even animals that hibernate don't pile on the pounds before winter arrives. A furry creature that became obese would be killed and eaten long before it retired to its burrow. Their strategy for surviving winter is not to put on weight, but to slow down their metabolisms so they require less food and stay alive and healthy throughout the period of hibernation.

To some extent nature keeps an animal's obesity level in check through balancing the availability and scarcity of food. But there are times when food is plentiful, and still animals in the wild don't get fat. It follows therefore that animals in the wild have an internal mechanism that tells them when to eat and when to stop eating in order to maintain themselves in the optimum physical condition for their survival. Somehow they know that if they were to eat too much they would become vulnerable, and so they don't do it.

What is also interesting is that NONE of the members of a particular species of animal in the wild get fat. You do not see some lions in the jungle with a weight problem and others who don't. Of course, there are genetic differences between animals of the same species. For example, elephants do not all grow to the same height. One horse may be taller or more muscular than another. But it remains a fact that despite differences in height and muscularity etc., there are no differences between wild animals of ANY species when it comes to obesity.

Animals in captivity, however, do sometimes get fat. They share the same genetic code as those in the wild – it is their behaviour or lifestyle that is different. So it appears that if you take an animal out of its natural environment and cause it to lead an unnatural life, the mechanism for controlling obesity can be overridden, with the inevitable health consequences.

But what about humans? We differ in terms of our height, muscularity and hair colour etc., but we also have enormous differences in our body fat percentages. Are some of us following unnatural lifestyles, or have we undergone a genetic mutation that has changed our fundamental nature? We are highly developed beings – could we have evolved in a different way to other species?

If Darwin's Theory of Evolution is correct, (the survival of the fittest), then it follows that any genetic changes occurring within our species would always be advantageous to us. How could getting fat be beneficial to our survival?

We know the problems that gaining weight causes, (high blood pressure, diabetes, increased risk of cancer, heart disease etc.), and so there is no doubt that it is unhealthy for us and therefore prejudices our survival. It could also be argued that it is unhelpful to the survival of our species in that it makes it harder for us to find a mate. There is simply no logic in us mutating in this way.

But there is also another piece of evidence that tells us there cannot be a genetic factor in the rise of obesity: The change is occurring too fast.

Newspapers are full of the latest surveys telling us the western world is getting fatter. We constantly hear horror stories about overweight children with obesity-related ailments normally found in people much older. Airlines are making their seats wider to accommodate the expanding girths of their passengers. When you compare the average body fat percentages of people thirty years ago with people today, the difference is staggering. And one thing we know about genetic mutations is that they cannot occur in such a short space of time.

This rules them out as a potential cause

of the rise in obesity.

So what can we conclude from this?

1. All species of animals living in their natural environment remain slim – the state that is most advantageous to their survival.

2. Despite differences in height, muscularity, etc., EVERY MEMBER of an animal species in the wild remains slim. In other words, when it comes to obesity, there is no difference between them.

3. Only animals in captivity (leading unnatural lives) become fat.

4. According to Darwin's Theory of Evolution, genetic changes will only occur if they help a species to survive.

5. The rise in the rate of obesity in humans has no benefit for us, and has occurred too quickly for genetic mutation to be the cause.

All this is wonderful news! It shows us that an overweight person has essentially the same genetic makeup as a naturally slim person. It means that in terms of obesity, none of us are trapped by our genetic inheritance, only our behaviour, *and that is something we can change.* Putting it another way, whether you are morbidly obese, or slightly overweight, you are perfectly capable of changing your body. Slimness is our natural state of being, the one that is most beneficial to our survival. Becoming slim can only be a question of identifying and following behaviour that corresponds to our nature. And if it is natural to us it can't be hard to follow, can it?

Having understood this, I knew I could never again look at a naturally slim person and tell myself they were, "just born lucky." I realised that the differences between overweight and slim people could only be caused by behavioural or psychological factors.

Which led me to the next question:

5

Why Do Humans Behave Unnaturally?

There is an obvious difference between animals and human beings: Animals never act against their nature, humans often do.

How can this be?

In considering this I realised that part of the reason why humans sometimes act unnaturally is simply because we can.

We have a unique form of consciousness that gives us the ability to devise new patterns of behaviour that we think will be beneficial. Unfortunately we are not infallible, and often we fail to predict the long-term consequences of the behaviour patterns we adopt. However, the same mental ability that allows us to act in a way that is against our nature can also be used to bring us back on track.

But changing unnatural behaviour is not just a matter of identifying it. It is not that simple. We are constantly reminded that we should eat less and exercise more – but still most of us can do nothing about it. Our resolve disappears the moment we are offered a large slice of chocolate cake.

But why is it so difficult to eat the way we all know we should?

In an attempt to find the cause of our desire to overeat, I looked back at my own eating history to try to find out when and why it all started.

6

The Start Of Overeating

One thing I remember from my childhood is the excitement I felt whenever my mother baked a cake. It wasn't the thought of biting into a large slice of jam sponge cake that got me salivating (although a slice of warm cake fresh from the oven was always irresistible) – it was the thought of licking the mixing bowl clean. There was something about that sweet-tasting sugary mixture that really did it for me. It seemed to be a shame to put it in the oven at all.

When I was ten years old I stayed at the house of a friend who shared my cake-mix fixation, and I remember getting up in the middle of the night and making a huge bowl of it, which we scoffed down in record time before washing everything up and destroying the evidence.

I remember visiting my grandparents on Sunday evenings and being presented with a feast of food, including homemade bread, cakes and trifles. I would never miss out on the chance to indulge myself. After filling my stomach until it was painful I would slump down into an armchair, unable to move.

But I was never accused of being a glutton. Eating huge quantities of food was encouraged –
it was the sign of a "healthy appetite." To my grandparents, eating so much of their food was a compliment to their cooking. It is possible that at times I may have been told, "Eat everything on your plate before you leave the table," but if I was I can't remember. In my case I don't think that instruction was ever necessary.

And yet despite all this eating, I was never

obese as a young child. It wasn't until I was twelve years old that I first became aware things might be going in the wrong direction.

When playing football at school, the games teacher made a comment about my weight, which jolted me into an uncomfortable state of self-consciousness, and I began to wonder if I was getting fat. I had never been taunted in the playground about my weight – but I had probably put on a few pounds, and the thought of getting tubby left me frightened and embarrassed. But however worrying the thought of encroaching obesity may have been, it didn't stop me from overeating.

At this same school lunch was served in a dining room with rows of tables, at which would sit twelve boys. A 'Server' was elected to go into the kitchens and bring out trays of food to the waiting gaggle of students. I can still remember the wonderful smell of roast beef, roast lamb, and rice pudding for desert. Not all the boys had enormous appetites, and there was usually plenty left over for a second

The Key To Permanent Slimness

helping. A friend and I managed to get ourselves elevated to the position of 'Kitchen Monitor', which meant we stood in the kitchen and supervised the handing out of the trays of food to the Servers. We also supervised what happened to any food that might be brought back to the kitchen untouched, still on its serving trays.

This was binge time!

We could stuff ourselves at will with as much food as we could eat – and we did. Many times I walked out of the kitchen feeling bloated after an orgy of eating, and would find it almost impossible to keep awake during the afternoon lessons.

My unhealthy, destructive eating habits were becoming firmly established.

When I was fourteen years old I saw an advert on television for a food product that was supposed to help you slim. The advert asked the viewer to try to "pinch more than an inch" of fat on their stomachs. If they could they needed to buy the product.

A friend of mine lifted his shirt, pinched his stomach, and challenged me to do the same. I knew only too well what the embarrassing outcome would be, but I could hardly refuse such a challenge, could I? Of course I pinched more than an inch. Infuriatingly, he couldn't. Was I destined to become fat? Did I really eat too much? It didn't feel like I did. It all seemed grossly unfair.

Many of these early memories are painful, which is why they have stuck in my mind for so long. In looking back at them, I did not find one particular event that caused me to start overeating. It seems that in my case it was a creeping habit that became established over several years.

However, the process of revisiting those early memories was extremely useful to me, and raised the level of consciousness I had of my eating habits, which is a necessary requirement for getting power over any habit and changing it.

I recommend that you spend some time

The Key To Permanent Slimness

now thinking back to your earliest recollections of overeating and how the habit became embedded in your lifestyle.

After enduring the embarrassment and discomfort of an expanding waistline, the time eventually arrives when we decide we really must do something about it. And what is the miracle cure we all inevitably turn to?

Dieting!

We are promised by countless books, TV advertisements, billboards, and now the Internet, that the latest fad diet will cure our weight problems forever, leaving us as thin and sexually attractive as the models who smile out at us, beckoning us to join them in their slim and happy world.

Is there a magic diet out there that will save us all from obesity?

Let's see what we can learn from my own dieting history.

7

My Dieting Phase.

Years ago the only way to diet I knew of was to restrict the calories I ate. Some clever scientist had worked out how much food I was supposed to eat, and as long as I stuck to the regime I would lose weight and get slim. Great. But this was a non-starter for me – I enjoyed my food too much. I knew I would never stick to the tiny portions I was supposed to eat, and the idea of spending the rest of my life eating salads and crispbread was about as appealing as having a tooth drilled. So I refused to even try.

But when I was in my late twenties, I heard of something called Food Combining, and it seemed to be the answer to my prayers. The basis of the diet was to avoid eating proteins and complex carbohydrates at the same time. In other words I could eat fish or meat with salad or vegetables, but couldn't have potatoes or rice with it. Pasta, rice, and potatoes were not forbidden – I could eat them at another time, along with salad or vegetables. I just had to choose whether I was going to eat a carbohydrate meal or a protein meal, and stick to it. Fruit was to be eaten on its own.

What could be simpler than that?

Apparently, carbohydrates and proteins require different conditions for digestion – one alkaline, the other acidic. It you eat the two types of food together they "fight each other" and the digestive process is slowed down. Separating the food is supposed to help your digestion and cause you to lose weight.

I set off to follow the diet religiously, confident that I would soon have a slim fit-looking body. At first everything went well and I began to lose weight and feel better. I was eating more healthily too, increasing my intake of salads and vegetables, even making my own wholemeal bread, (which was delicious when lightly buttered). I was supposed to eat one protein-based meal, one carbohydrate-based meal, and one meal consisting of neutral foods (salads and vegetables) per day, but I soon ran into difficulties with this because I found the protein-based meals to be unsatisfying, (a steak just didn't fill me up as much as a large baked potato dripping with butter). Before long I was eating carbohydrate-based meals almost exclusively. And then there was the problem of eating out.

In theory this shouldn't have been a problem. I just had to stick to protein-based meals and tell the waiter to replace the potatoes with more salad or vegetables. Easy, right? Well, it was at first. But after a few weeks on the diet I visited a restaurant, chose a protein-based dish, enjoyed it – and then the waiter slipped the desert menu into my hand!

Was I to spend the rest of my life denying

myself the mouth-watering creations that lay before me? Not likely. The lure of a crème caramel was always too tempting for me to resist, so I had one, and then drove away from the restaurant feeling depressed, beating myself up for my lack of willpower.

When I arrived home I reasoned that having broken the diet I might as well treat myself to something really bad. After all, I could start the diet again in the morning and do it properly next time, couldn't I?

A whole packet of biscuits later I tumbled into bed and in the morning came to the conclusion that Food Combining was not for me.

I tried the Atkins Diet next. This one sounded great – no limits on how much I could eat – just leave out the carbohydrates and fill myself up with as much protein and fat as I wanted. Bacon and eggs for breakfast, roast chicken and cheese for lunch, cheese omelettes with more bacon for dinner – fantastic!

I began to lose weight, but after a few

weeks I craved the clean taste of fruit, and my constant bad breath, (which came with the diet), wasn't exactly conducive to social interactions.

I became seriously bored by the food I was eating, and the thought of spending my whole life on the Atkins diet was too much to bear.

When I broke the diet the weight came rushing back. It was as if my body had been crying out for carbohydrates, and the moment it got wind of any it converted them to fat, storing them away on my body like a squirrel might store nuts for winter.

Then came the Zone Diet. To me this seemed to be a kind of "Atkins Lite." The carbohydrate quantities were higher, and I could eat more fruit. But, I had to balance out the carbohydrate, protein, and fat proportions of each meal to a precise formula, and adhere to strict quantity restrictions based on my size and activity level. I became terrified of breaking the rules – so much so that at one point I was eating nothing but their own pre-prepared meals, which had the prescribed food mix.

I lost weight initially, but the rigidity of the diet was unsustainable, and I couldn't envisage spending the rest of my life weighing out my food. Eventually I became highly suspicious of the need to balance out the food types because the diet's quantity restrictions meant I was only eating 1800 calories a day, and at that level of calorific intake I would lose weight no matter what I ate, wouldn't I?

I binned the Zone Diet along with the others I had tried. Of course I didn't stop dieting. I continued looking for the elusive super-diet that would solve my weight problem once and for all. I tried the Carbohydrate Addicts Diet, the G.I. Diet, and others – all with the same lack of success.

It was a sad and sorry period of my life, littered with partial successes and eventual failures, and at the end of it all I was no slimmer, just more aware than ever that there were people in this world who didn't have to go through all this misery.

The Key To Permanent Slimness

Why was I so different?

Now spend some time reflecting on your own diet history. Remember how you felt when you were on each diet, and how you felt when you eventually gave it up.

We are about to learn some important lessons from this and discover why ALL diets fail.

8

Lessons From A History Of Dieting

I always achieved some weight loss, no matter which diet I was on, (even if I did put it all back on when I eventually stopped the programme). This seemed to indicate that they were "scientifically sound." But if so, why was I unable to stay on them for the long-term?

Of course it may have been that I just didn't have any willpower, but in other areas of my life I have achieved things that have required a great deal of willpower, and people who know me say I am a disciplined person. So why then would I not be able to stay on a diet, despite having been highly motivated for over thirty years to get rid of my excess fat? It didn't make any sense.

One summer, a family I know came to visit me, and I asked them about the new 'Detox' diet they had been on. They said the food tasted great and that they had felt better and lost weight, *while they were on it*. I asked them why, if they really did feel better eating this great tasting food and were losing weight, did they ever give it up? Just like me they were lost for an answer. It seems that there is something about diets that makes them impossible to stay on.

I thought long and hard about it, and then the answer came to me.

It doesn't matter which diet you follow, ALL are by their nature *restrictive* in some way. Whenever you deprive yourself of something, don't you increase your desire for it? Consciously fighting against something focuses your attention on whatever it is you are resisting. When you say to yourself that you will never eat chocolate again, don't you wake up dreaming of the stuff – desperate to rush out to the shops and buy a family-sized bar to stuff in your mouth? The act of denying yourself what you want merely stokes up your craving for it.

I asked myself why this should be, and then I remembered something from Newton's Third Law of Motion, which states: *For every action, there is an equal and opposite reaction.* In other words, the more you fight against eating a certain food, the bigger your desire for it becomes. You push harder and harder, but the opposing force (your craving) always matches your willpower, until eventually you are tired of fighting, give up resisting, and binge on whatever you were craving. And this will ALWAYS be the case because the laws of physics cannot be broken.

This was an important breakthrough in understanding why I had always failed to stay on a diet. In fact it is impossible to stay on them – they do not work in accordance with the fundamental nature of mankind.

Overeating is unnatural too. But how can we expect to cure the problems associated with one pattern of unnatural behaviour by substituting it with another that is equally unnatural? The idea is insane, and yet we've been trying to do it for years!

You will never see an animal in the jungle confront its prey and tell itself, "I mustn't eat meat today because it's a carbohydrate day." Nor will it question how many calories it has consumed that morning before deciding if it should eat something else. Animals in the wild just get on with the business of eating – and they don't get fat. Shouldn't it be like that for us too?

Well for some people it is!

Naturally slim people enjoy their food, eat what they want, stop when they are satisfied (with no sense of self-denial), and don't get fat. They are no different genetically to the rest of us, and so there is no reason why any of us should be unable to eat this way. It is the natural way for us to live.

But there is something else about dieting that is insidious and highly destructive to long-term slimness.

Whenever you follow a diet you are told to stick to the rules and guidelines, and nothing else. But these formulas exist EXTERNALLY to you. They have no connection to your own intelligent internal mechanism (hunger feelings), which tell you when and how much you need to eat. Animals in the wild and humans who are naturally slim always listen to their internal voice – it is the ONLY valid authority on what and when they should eat. By concentrating solely on the guidelines of any diet you are distancing yourself from the thing you need to connect with if you are ever going to eat naturally and become permanently slim.

This is extremely damaging!

When I grasped this I realised that not only were diets unnatural, and therefore impossible to stay on, they were also actively

The Key To Permanent Slimness

DESTRUCTIVE to my long-term weight loss, and for years had connived in keeping me fat.

It really was the end of dieting for me – and it should be for you too.

But if diets aren't the cure for obesity, then what is? Maybe the answer can be found in another traditional remedy.

Can exercise offer us some hope?

Let's take a look.

9

Is Exercise The Cure?

We are constantly bombarded with advertisements telling us that some new exercise fad will give us a freshly toned, slim body. And yet the world is getting fatter.

I spent a long time trying to unravel why this might be and I realised that to avoid confusion it is necessary to look at the potential benefits of exercise separately.

There is no doubt that regular exercise will have a dramatic effect on a person's health and fitness. It is beyond question, and so not worth dwelling on for the purposes of this book.

The Key To Permanent Slimness

However, in the western world humans require comparatively little physical fitness for survival, and the reason why most people embark on an exercise programme is to lose weight rather than to get fit. (Of course, if exercising could make you slim your health would improve because more health problems are caused by obesity than anything else.)

So how effective is exercise for losing weight?

I have tried to get slim by exercising many times, but it has never worked for me. In purely scientific terms, to lose weight we must burn more calories than we ingest. But given that one pound of fat = 3500 calories, and thirty minutes of jogging burns approximately 300 calories, to lose an appreciable amount of fat one would have to exercise for a period of time that just isn't practical for most of us. This is the case even when taking into account the fat burning effect of the body's increased metabolic rate, which remains elevated after exercising has stopped. And of course, however much you exercise you still won't lose weight if afterwards you eat more calories than you have burned off. Personally I always seemed to feel ravenously hungry after going for a run, and because I had exercised I would tell myself, "Hey, you can have a little treat today!"

Sad but true.

When looking for the most efficient way of losing weight, if we compare exercising against reducing our food intake, cutting down on what we eat always wins. It doesn't take up any time or interrupt our daily schedule, and you don't need any special equipment to do it. Yes, I know it isn't easy to cut down on your food. You and I have tried and failed at it many times. But in purely scientific terms, when it comes to losing weight it is much more efficient than exercise.

We could spend time going into all the psychological reasons why we don't stick at exercise, but we don't have to. For the most part they are similar to why we don't stay on diets, (discipline, willpower etc.) But there is another psychological factor we have to consider that is unique to exercising: A rotund body just doesn't look good in Lycra!

Sitting on an exercise bike with your buttocks hanging down on either side of the saddle is not good for your self-esteem – especially when there is a toned Adonis on the bike next to you!

Fear of looking stupid is probably the biggest deterrent to going to the gym, and is also a reason why you rarely see obese people out running.

Most people will not show themselves in a jogging kit until their weight is low enough for them to feel comfortable being seen in one. People are more inclined to exercise WHEN they have become slim, rather than use it as a means of losing weight.

What we can conclude from this is that exercise alone will never make us slim. It takes too long to burn up the calories, and the resistance to staying on an exercise programme is too great for most people, particularly those who are overweight. Which is why some people hire a Personal Trainer with the attitude of a Drill Sergeant to bully them into doing it.

Does this sound like a natural way of life to you?

Here is an astonishing fact: None of the naturally slim people I studied when writing this book took any exercise at all! They didn't run, they didn't go to the gym, or play sport. They were slim already, so why should they bother to exercise?

Soon you will know the key to permanent slimness and will be able to choose to exercise or play sport for health and fitness reasons, or for the sheer enjoyment of it, rather that to lose weight.

10

Saying Goodbye To Traditional Thinking

We have just applied some logical thinking to the two traditional 'cures' for obesity. By now you should see that all diets are unnatural, impossible to follow and are *actively destructive* to your goal of becoming permanently slim.

We have also looked at exercise and concluded that for psychological reasons it is hard to either start or keep doing it – particularly when you are overweight. We have compared its potential for making us slim against the time and effort required to achieve any significant weight loss, and found it to be very inefficient.

You may be asking yourself, "If not either of these two traditional approaches, then what is the solution to becoming slim?"

Short of any alternative it is tempting to continue along the same old routes, even if they have never taken you where you wanted to go. But remember this: *A key will always stay hidden if you keep looking in the wrong place.*

At this point it is important that you keep your mind open to new thinking because we are about to turn conventional 'wisdom' on its head.

Bear in mind that for thousands of years human beings thought the Earth was a stationary object in space. Then Gallileo came up with the idea that the Earth was spinning, and that once a year it revolved around the sun. What followed was a giant leap in man's understanding, and things were never the same again. A similar shift in thinking is about to propel you to a life of permanent slimness.

11

A Closer Look At Food Cravings

After realising that no diet or exercise programme would ever make me slim, I knew that if I was ever going to find a solution to the problem I had to get right down to the root of what I experienced whenever I overate.

There were times when I could restrain myself and eat sensibly, such as when I started a new diet, but the cravings always returned, and when they did I was in binge-mode, and the only thing that interested me was stuffing food in my mouth as quickly as possible to experience the emotional high overeating gave me.

The Key To Permanent Slimness

My desire for that high was drug-like in its intensity. I can think of no other way to describe it. I remember once telling a naturally slim person what it felt like to buy a packet of biscuits, a sponge cake, or a custard-based desert (my favourite), and scoff the lot down in one sitting. I told her that in moments like these my desire was so strong that it felt as if I wanted to SUBMERGE myself in the food – to swim in it almost. Needless to say she gave me a horrified look. It was quite a picture.

My food orgies would continue until my stomach cried out in pain, at which point I would stop eating, my energy level would plunge and I would fall asleep, only to wake up full of guilt and self-loathing after becoming aware of what I had done.

Think for a moment how you feel when you overindulge, whether it be on fried potatoes, chocolate, or anything else. Don't you behave like a drug addict needing a fix?

But the question I kept asking myself was *why* did I do this, when I knew in my rational moments how destructive it was to my health and my general sense of wellbeing?

Eventually I was struck by something that seemed to be significant:

When I was in binge-mode, the rational part of my brain was shut down.

It didn't matter what I knew regarding healthy, normal eating – that knowledge was not available to me. It was buried beneath my desire for the endorphin rush I craved so much when I overate.

But the eating habits of the naturally slim are rational. It follows therefore, that the logical part of their brain remains engaged whenever they are confronted with food.

I knew that if I were ever to get slim I would have to find a way of keeping the rational part of my brain engaged when I ate.

I was sure this had to be an important part of the key to permanent slimness.

12

The Dual Aspect of Eating

There are two aspects to eating: the physical and the psychological. We can never separate them entirely, but it is useful to look at them independently when trying to understand the secret of the naturally slim.

The physical aspect is relatively straightforward. We need to eat to survive and when our bodies determine that we need food we are sent an "I'm hungry" signal, which is unpleasant, and we search around for something to eat to rid ourselves of our hunger sensations.

This hunger signal is an important part of

our design, and works FOR us by making sure we are topped up with fuel in the form of energy-giving food. It would be dangerous to cut ourselves off from these sensations entirely.

The psychological aspect of eating relates to the pleasure we derive from it. When we eat foods we like our taste buds send signals to our brains, which release powerful opiate-like chemicals called endorphins, giving us a high, and it is this high that we crave when we go on a food binge. In fact we are all drug addicts – addicted to the chemicals produced inside our brains.

Of course the pleasure we get from eating is entirely natural – or else why would we have been designed in a way that allows us to enjoy it so much? The high we experience is crucial for our psychological wellbeing and also aids our physical survival in that (as is the case with sex) because it is so enjoyable we are encouraged to do it, and so our species continues to thrive.

If getting pleasure from food is natural for us, then we can conclude that it would be unnatural to do anything that diminishes the pleasure of eating. Which is great news. It means that in order to live a natural life, we must ALWAYS enjoy our food.

Releasing the endorphins in our brains is crucial to our satisfaction and one of the ways we do this is by eating. Which led me to wonder why, if it is natural for all of us to enjoy the high we get from our food, do the naturally slim feel no compulsion to overeat? Could it be that they get their endorphin rush in a different way and enjoy their food less than the rest of us? If this were the case it would be impossible for me to prove. I would never be able to experience what someone else felt when they were eating, and so would be unable to make a comparison.

But I didn't have to.

I realised that if this theory were true it would mean that the rapid rise in obesity had been caused by physical changes in the taste buds of those who gain weight. This would amount to a genetic mutation of some kind, and as we know, it is impossible for this to be the cause for reasons we have already discussed.

I had another reason to disregard any theory about naturally slim people getting less pleasure from eating than the rest of us:

The naturally slim people I studied whilst writing this book enjoyed their food!

One of them was a cordon bleu cook who loved to prepare exotic meals, and whose hobby was finding new restaurants to try. Another was fanatical about spicy food – Thai and Asian in particular – so the theory just didn't stack up.

Struggling to find an answer, I looked at the problem from another angle and wondered if overweight people might in some way get pleasure from overfilling their stomachs. But this made no sense. Where is the pleasure in stuffing yourself until you are in pain?

However, it struck me that in an extreme

case it might be possible for a person to gorge on food past the point of physical pain, and get *psychological* satisfaction from it (albeit of a perverse nature), if the pleasure came not from the taste of the food, but through the act of getting as much of it inside their stomach as possible – an extreme form of greed or gluttony. Not a pleasant thought. But I was sure I had witnessed this on at least one occasion.

The answer to why naturally slim people stayed that way effortlessly, while those who overate were slaves to their food cravings continued to elude me. I knew that even if I could come up with the answer there was no guarantee I would somehow be able to change myself and become like them. There seemed to be no logical line of thought that lead me to where I wanted to go.

Eventually I realised that trying to follow a logical straight-line train of thought had kept me in ignorance. What I needed was a lateral leap in thinking. And then I had my "Eureka" moment, and everything became clear.

13

Revealing The Secret

How would it be if we could somehow harness the drug-like power that food has over us, and use it to make us STOP eating, rather than eat too much?

Let me put it another way:

Wouldn't it be amazing if we could take our craving for the food we love, flip it around, and use it to make us eat LESS?

Think about this for a moment.

We know how irresistible our cravings are –powerful enough to overcome our willpower every time. If it were possible to harness this power and have it work FOR us, rather than against us, wouldn't we have to most potent weapon ever devised in the fight against obesity? We would be using our own naturally occurring mood-elevating super-drug to make us slim!

Sounds impossible?

Well, believe it or not, this is exactly what the naturally slim do – without even realising it! And after finishing this book it is exactly what you are going to do. I am going to show you how it's done.

But before that, it's important for you to understand how I came to have this leap in thinking – my "Eureka" moment.

When talking about someone who is overweight, people often say: "Oh, he enjoys his food too much." It suddenly occurred to me that this 'wisdom' is completely wrong, and in fact the complete opposite is true:

People who are overweight don't enjoy their food enough!

I'll explain:

There is essentially no genetic difference between those people who are naturally slim and those who gain weight. Also, both groups of people are the same psychologically in that they need to experience the high they get from eating food they enjoy.

However, the naturally slim get their pleasurable high from food AT THE SAME MOMENT they relieve themselves from their feelings of hunger. Which means they never have a psychological need to keep on eating after their hunger has been satisfied.

Those who overeat, on the other hand, do not achieve psychological satisfaction at the same moment their hunger disappears – and so have to keep on eating until their endorphins are released.

It follows therefore that the naturally slim are able to extract MORE pleasurable sensations from a given amount of food than the overweight, and because of this have no desire to eat more than they need. Because the physical and psychological needs of the naturally slim are satisfied simultaneously, a natural balance is achieved. So:

The difference between the naturally slim and the overweight is the amount of pleasure each gets from a given amount of food.

This means that if we were to find a way of bringing on the endorphin rush sooner in those who are overweight, they could eliminate their need to overeat, and would be able to satisfy their psychological and physical needs simultaneously, establishing a natural balance, just like that of the naturally slim.

So how could this be achieved?

It is the pleasurable sensation of taste that causes the endorphins to be released. So to encourage them to be released earlier, all we have to do is find a way to increase the sensation of taste we experience from a given amount of food!

It all sounded so incredibly simple. And if it really were the path to permanent slimness, well, it wouldn't be too hard to follow, would it?

Bursting with enthusiasm to see if this

idea could deliver the dramatic changes I hoped it would, I immediately put it to the test.

What followed was one of the most amazing periods of my life. After thirty years of battling to get slim and always succumbing to my desire to binge, my whole experience of eating changed. Suddenly every mouthful of food seemed to have a fuller, stronger flavour and for the first time in my life I was TRULY enjoying my food. I seemed to be more connected to my hunger sensations, more aware of when they started and when they stopped, and the moment they had gone I was able to stop eating easily, without summoning up ANY willpower whatsoever.

I was constantly amazed by how little I needed to eat to feel satisfied and I realised just how much I had been overeating throughout my life.

In the mirror, I could see myself getting slimmer, and my trousers became loser. For eight weeks I deliberately avoided the scales, but then, so I could measure exactly what I had achieved, I did weigh myself, and found that my weight had dropped to the second lowest it had ever been through dieting – and I hadn't been on a diet!

Had I gone through a permanent change or was this temporary, just like in the early days of starting a new diet? Would I eventually resort to my old habit of bingeing? Although I felt none of my usual cravings, I wondered if I might be tipped over the edge by one of the foods I had always found irresistible.

Remember those sweet-tasting custard-based deserts I mentioned earlier? I would often buy them in a pack of four and wolf the lot down in five minutes. To test myself I bought some – but this time things were different. I opened one and began to eat it, enjoying its wonderful flavour (and it seemed to taste even better than before), but after eating just half of one of the deserts, I put the tub in the fridge along with the other three and shut the door. *There was no need for any willpower.* I felt completely satisfied. One week later I eventually finished the last of the tubs. What had previously taken me five minutes to eat had lasted for seven days!

Now I knew things had changed!

More weeks passed, and still I felt no compulsion to binge. My energy level rose higher than it had ever been (it was as if I had thrown off some dark cloud that had been hanging over me all my life) and I no longer felt the need to sleep after a meal. I was living and eating the way I was born to – the way of the naturally slim, and having experienced this new way of being I knew I would never go back to my old habits of overeating and gaining weight. *I had found the key to permanent slimness!*

And the good news is that there is nothing unusual about me. I am no different to anyone else who has struggled to get slim and been constantly unhappy with their body shape. So it will work for you too, no matter if you are slightly overweight, or morbidly obese.

I shared the secret with someone who had a similar diet and weight-gaining history to me.

The Key To Permanent Slimness

As the weeks went by he phoned me from time to time, always amazed by how little he was eating, how good he felt, and how he had lost all desire to overeat. He felt as if someone had cast a magic spell on him. He told me a relative had stayed with him for a week, and in that time they had eaten out twice a day, every day. At the end of the week he was astounded to find that rather than gaining five pounds (as would normally be the case), he had actually lost two!

It was great news, but not altogether surprising. I knew this would work for everyone, because it is completely at one with both the physical AND psychological nature of mankind.

In wondering why this secret hadn't been discovered before, it occurred to me that it was a bit like seeing a magic trick performed by a great conjurer. It looks amazing, but it's impossible to see how it's done because your attention is always drawn to the wrong place. Of course, when the trick is explained to you it seems so incredibly simple.

However the difference in this case is that the conjurers are the naturally slim, and even they don't realise the trick they are performing!

You now understand the THEORY of the key to permanent slimness - but this it is not enough. To change your life and become one of the naturally slim you must take the practical steps necessary to EXPERIENCE the power of it (which only takes about two days!).

So let's look at how you do that.

14

Practical Guide To Changing Your Eating Experience

Basic Principles

Everything I am going to tell you is designed to give you a different eating experience. It is very detailed, but don't let that put you off. The more you incorporate these suggestions into your eating habits the better your experience will be. After a short period of time it will all become second nature to you.

If we are to eat naturally we must make our sensation of hunger the SOLE guide to when and how much we eat. This may sound simple, but it's not. We have developed set meal times called breakfast, lunch and dinner, and when we arrive at our usual time for one of these we tend to eat, whether we are hungry or not, reacting unconsciously like one of Pavlov's dogs.

Dieticians trot out the advice that we should always have a substantial breakfast and that it is the "most important meal of the day." *Do not fall for this nonsense.* If you wake up and you feel hungry, then of course you should eat something. But if you are not feeling hungry why put food in your mouth? Your lack of hunger means your body is telling you that you don't need any food at this time. To eat when you are not hungry, just because some 'expert' says it's a 'good idea', is damaging to your goal of developing the correct relationship with your body's hunger mechanism.

But if we are to abandon set meal times and eat only when we are hungry, there are two issues that must be addressed:

The Key To Permanent Slimness

The first is the FEAR of becoming hungry. Often we eat when we are not hungry to stave off possible feelings of hunger later on. Remember, you can eat WHENEVER you are hungry. And that means that even if only an hour has passed since you last ate, you can still have something else.

This is ABSOLUTELY CRUCIAL to your success. You must establish this idea firmly in your mind. If you don't you will never be able to stop eating at the precise moment your hunger disappears, and will always cram in a little more 'just in case.'

The second issue is a practical one. What do you do if you get up without feeling hungry, leave home for work without eating anything, and then feel hungry at 11.00am?

The answer is, of course, you eat something – but this means you must have something to hand. If not there is a danger your hunger will spiral out of control, which will make you binge.

You will not have to carry food around

with you forever – just in the early stages of changing your eating habits.

How hungry you feel – and nothing else – must determine not only WHEN you eat, but also HOW MUCH you eat. Let's suppose it is now 11.00am and you are feeling hungry, so you take out a sandwich. How much of it will you eat – all of it, or half of it?

Most people wouldn't give this a moment's thought. You are hungry, you are having a sandwich, the sandwich is whatever size it is, and so you just eat it. But some sandwiches are small and delicate; others are made from a baguette with great lumps of filling. *The point is that the size of the sandwich may or may not bear any relation to the level of hunger you are feeling.* If you need all of it to eliminate your hunger, then of course you should go ahead and eat it. But maybe half would be enough?

This is an important part of the key to permanent slimness. Soon you will become aware that we are programmed to eat what is in front of us, rather than what our bodies are telling us we need.

The same principal applies wherever and whenever you eat. At home you might make a meal that is too big for your needs – and you certainly will when you first start to eat naturally. But when you do, there's no problem. Put whatever you haven't eaten in the fridge and use it for a snack later.

In restaurants portion sizes vary enormously. Sometimes we are served dishes that are small and artistically prepared; other times we are served a mountain of food. But what has the portion size got to do with the level of hunger you feel in your stomach?

You may say to yourself, "I've paid for it, so it would be a shame to waste it," but the bill will be the same at the end of the meal whether you eat it all, or just half of it. However, if you continue to eat after your hunger feelings have disappeared you will pay for it twice – once financially, and secondly, through the fat you add to your waistline.

Remember you are there to enjoy the chef's cooking, not damage yourself by eating an unnatural quantity of it, and if you feel hungry when you get home you can always have something else.

Some of you may be thinking this is all well and good, but stopping eating when there is all that tempting food in front of me is impossible. Don't worry. By the time you have finished reading this book you will realise why this will no longer be an issue for you.

It is a good idea to give yourself a 'hunger-percentage-rating' before you begin your meal. Something between 10 and 100%. Then as you eat, be conscious of when your hunger disappears, and notice how much you still have left on your plate. You will be as surprised as I was by just how little you need to feel satisfied, and will come to see how much you have been overeating throughout your life. After a few days you will become better connected with your body's hunger mechanism, and will begin to make smaller meals.

The Key To Permanent Slimness

If you are preparing food for your family it is a good idea (whenever possible) to put the food in serving bowls, rather than directly onto the plates. This allows people to take only what THEY feel they need, and so encourages them to begin eating naturally. Of course if they haven't taken enough, they can always take some more later on.

Choose the foods you really like. Do not deprive yourself of something you have a real desire for. If you do you will eventually develop a craving for it and will be tempted to binge. Remember it is not the *type* of food you eat, but the *quantity* of it in relation to the calories you burn off that determines whether you lose weight or not. Naturally slim people eat what they want, when they want – even chocolate – but they enjoy the taste of one or two squares of it, rather than stuff themselves with a whole family-sized bar in an unconscious eating-frenzy.

The Key To Permanent Slimness

Mental preparation

Remember your goal is to maximise the stimulation of your taste buds, so you get the pleasurable endorphin release in your brain at the earliest possible moment. To help you achieve this, just before you begin to eat, tell yourself:

"I am a food TASTER, not a food binger."

THIS IS VITAL TO YOUR SUCCESS. You must keep your attention on TASTING your food whenever you eat. Most of us think about something else at meal times – problems at work, relationship issues etc. Having your mind elsewhere makes it impossible to enjoy the taste of your food, delays the endorphin rush, and so encourages you to keep on eating. Like sex, eating is a sensory pleasure, and if you don't have your mind on it you can't expect to enjoy it.

Now remind yourself that YOU, AND YOU ALONE are in control of what you eat, and that you will stop eating the moment your hunger has gone, safe in the knowledge that you can always eat something else later, WHENEVER you feel the need. Do not allow portion size to control your body shape.

Let's look now at the physical business of eating and what we can do to extract the maximum amount of taste from our food.

<u>Eating</u>

We have on average 10,000 taste buds in our mouth, and ABOLUTELY NONE in our stomachs. This seemingly unexceptional piece of information is very important.

When I was in binge-mode the only thing in my mind was shovelling lumps of food in my mouth and getting them down to my stomach as fast as I could. Experiencing the TASTE of the food was never paramount in my mind. Taste was just a pleasant by-product of the eating process. After realising just how important experiencing taste is to staying slim,

I became aware of how destructive this had been to my goal of losing weight.

An obvious requirement for getting the maximum amount of taste from a given amount of food is to keep it in your mouth for as long as possible. The instant it becomes detached from your taste buds it loses all of its potential to satisfy you psychologically. I realised that by swallowing my food too quickly I had probably been missing out on 80% of the potential satisfaction available to me.

Think about this for a moment.

It means that if I could extract 100% of the taste sensations from my food I would become psychologically satisfied after eating only a fifth of what I normally ate! What a difference this would make to my food cravings!

I am now going to give you the guidelines I followed to get the maximum amount of taste from my food. At first they will feel strange, and you might feel stupid concentrating so hard on something as simple as eating. But

The Key To Permanent Slimness

remind yourself that NOT thinking about eating (turning off your rational mind) has caused you to get fat. You won't have to concentrate like this forever – just until these guidelines become second nature to you – and they will – because they will increase the pleasure you get from eating and make you slim. And that can't be bad can it?

1. Take small mouthfuls. When your mouth is full the desire to swallow some of your food soon becomes overwhelming, and once it is on its way to your stomach it has lost all its potential to stimulate your taste buds. This is a "waste of taste." If you are feeling very hungry – relax! Remind yourself that the food will be inside your stomach soon enough, and those hunger pangs will disappear.

    2. Chew your food slowly. By this I mean at a fraction of your normal speed. Imagine you are eating in a slow-motion movie. This is going to feel strange at first but it will pay huge dividends. When you chew slowly you give your

food time to release all its flavours and allow yourself the opportunity to fully experience them.

3. When your food is chewed it becomes moist and liquefies. Much of the taste can be found in these juices, and an effective way to get the most enjoyment from your food is to swallow ONLY them, while retaining the solid food in your mouth for further chewing and flavour release. Do not swallow the solid part of the food until all its flavour has been extracted and enjoyed. You might find this a little difficult at first, but I advise you to practice it. You will be amazed by how much more enjoyment you get from each mouthful.

4. Put your knife and fork down after taking each mouthful. Do not begin to load up your fork again until you have swallowed all the food in your mouth AND HAVE TAKEN A MOMENT TO APPRECIATE ITS TASTE! This has two benefits: Firstly, it gives your food time to get to your stomach and for you to notice when your feelings of hunger have been eliminated.

The Key To Permanent Slimness

This enables you to stop eating when you are satisfied without consuming more food than you need. Secondly, it keeps your rational mind activated. You may remember I said earlier that I realised it would be impossible for me to binge if my rational mind were always engaged when I ate. When you look inward to monitor how hungry you feel AND how great your food tastes, you are EVALUATING your feelings, and the evaluation of a feeling is a left-brained, rational thing.

5. When you are eating do not do anything else. Turn off the television and concentrate on what you are doing. You cannot enjoy a sensory experience if your mind is distracted from it. This is the time to derive maximum pleasure from eating and nothing else. After a week or two you won't have to be so strict with the rules, but you are in the early stages of changing your habits, and it is important that you don't do anything that gets in the way of you having the same revelatory eating experience that I had. Your waistline

depends on it.

6. Halfway through your meal, stop for a moment and assess your level of hunger. You may find it has diminished rapidly and you need little or no more food to feel totally satisfied. You should already have experienced much enjoyment from your food and attained a level of psychological satisfaction. Do not stop eating if you still feel hungry. But if you *have* eaten enough, leave the rest of whatever is on your plate. You can always eat more later on if you feel the need.

7. Always eat sitting down. You will eat slower this way and will give yourself time to enjoy more of the flavour of your food.

IMPORTANT: The primary thing you must always focus on is TASTE. Experiencing more taste from your food is the sole reason why you must follow the physical actions listed above. THEY ARE NOT ENDS IN THEMSELVES!

I am emphasizing this because it is perfectly possible to take small mouthfuls, eat slowly, put your knife and fork down, etc., and still not taste your food – IF YOUR MIND IS ON SOMETHING ELSE. It is impossible for me to overstress this point.

Concentrating on taste whenever you eat is at the heart of the key to permanent slimness. If you ignore this advice you will almost certainly fail to experience what it is like to eat naturally, and will not succeed in becoming slim – so please don't!

It all sounds so simple doesn't it? No calorie counting, no restrictions on what, when, or how much you eat. No denying yourself anything – so no food cravings – and therefore no willpower required. As I have already said, after a short period of time the physical things listed above will become second nature to you. The early release of your endorphins will enable you to eat much less than before, whilst experiencing more pleasure from each meal. But before you put it into practice, here is some advice.

15

Some Helpful Advice

1. Think in terms of MOUTHFULS. Sometimes you will be served a mountain of food, and when you are, say to yourself, *"I am going to take a small mouthful of this, and really enjoy the taste."* When that mouthful is finished, take another, and continue eating, always monitoring your hunger level. The idea is that you *prescribe* yourself mouthfuls of food until your hunger has gone, which stops you thinking in terms of eating platefuls of food. Evaluating how many mouthfuls of food you need keeps your rational mind engaged and stops you bingeing.

2. Do not become obsessed with the scales. In fact I would advise you not to go on the scales at all in the early stages of learning to eat naturally. There are two reasons for this:

Firstly, you are not aiming to be any particular weight; you want to be slim. It doesn't matter what the scales say as long as your body shape is what you want it to be. To monitor how slim you are you need a mirror, not a set of scales.

Secondly, in the past when I was on a diet, I used the scales almost everyday. But weight loss is not always linear and can be affected by other things such as your body's level of hydration. There would inevitably be a time when the scales said I was heavier than the day before, and the resulting disappointment would sometimes make me give up the diet and go on a binge. So by weighing myself everyday I was setting myself up to fail. Don't make the same mistake.

3. Be patient. When you begin to eat naturally, the weight will drop off rapidly. But

The Key To Permanent Slimness

in your enthusiasm to "hurry the process along," you may start to leave the table before you are fully satisfied. This is a common mistake. Beware! If you deprive yourself you will develop a craving and will inevitably binge. The resulting feeling of hopelessness will be destructive to your goals, and it may take you some time to get back on track.

Remind yourself that you have been eating unnaturally for years and that you cannot realistically expect all your excess weight to drop off in only a couple of weeks. But it WILL disappear, I promise!

4. Prepare yourself to go off track once in a while - it will inevitably happen.

Some weeks after I began to eat naturally I was invited to dinner at the house of someone I didn't know very well. When I arrived I was offered a glass of wine, along with some tasty things to nibble on. After eating a few mouthfuls I realised my hunger pangs had completely disappeared – and we hadn't even got to the first course! What was I to do – eat nothing and offend my hosts, or eat something I knew I didn't need?

I ate something, of course, but tried to keep the quantity down to the minimum politeness allowed. Despite this I left the house feeling stuffed, and by the time I was halfway home a cloud of guilt hung over me and I questioned whether this way of eating would ever work for me. Fortunately I caught myself in the act of falling into this destructive trap and pulled myself out of it. I told myself that I was being ridiculous and that I would not allow one evening of overeating (brought about by social pressure) to determine my body shape for the rest of my life.

Something like this may, and almost certainly will happen to you. But once you have experienced how it feels to eat naturally these events will be rare.

5. Be prepared to be astounded by how little you need to eat to feel satisfied. I was constantly amazed by this. Being satisfied after eating only a fraction of what you previously

ate is a strange experience and can be difficult to get used to. At times you may even wonder if you are eating enough. But trust the intelligence of your body – it knows when and how much you need to eat. As long as you follow the advice in this book you will eat what is right for you, and will become slim naturally and permanently.

16

Some Final Thoughts

<u>An Alternative View</u>

In this book I have often used the analogy of heroin addiction to illustrate a point. If you are still having difficulty in understanding why something as simple as concentrating on taste works so well in losing weight, it is useful to take this analogy a little further and consider how heroin addicts try to kick their habit.

Just stopping "cold-turkey" is extremely difficult. Doctors know this, and so they often prescribe methadone as an alternative drug. In this way the addict is able to get a substitute fix and eventually replace his heroin habit. Similarly, smokers are often prescribed nicotine patches to help wean them off their harmful habit.

Overeaters also need their endorphin fix, which they eventually get after eating too much food. Kicking the habit of overeating by going "cold-turkey" is almost impossible. But with the key to permanent slimness the overeater can easily ditch his or her habit of eating too much by replacing it with a more satisfying alternative – a heightened experience of taste.

Thankfully this is perfectly natural and totally harmless!

Healthy Eating.

You may have noticed that until now I have avoided the subject of healthy eating. The reason is because this book is primarily about losing weight, and confusing these two issues is one of the reasons why the key to permanent slimness has remained hidden for so long.

The Key To Permanent Slimness

To get slim you must ingest fewer calories than you burn off – irrespective of which foods those calories come from. You could lose weight eating nothing but sugar and fat, providing you didn't eat much of it. But you don't need me to tell you this would not be a healthy diet and would soon give you problems. However, I have eaten healthily for most of my life, without losing weight – and it is a fact that obesity causes more health problems than does eating foods which are low in nutritional value.

In my experience it is better to establish the natural eating habits outlined in this book, bringing the habit of overeating under control, before looking at the relative health benefits of the foods you choose to eat.

Having said that, you can switch to healthier foods immediately if you choose to because eating naturally eliminates your food cravings instantly, leaving you free to make better food choices.

Personally, I found that the heightened experience of taste that comes from eating naturally meant that fruits, vegetables and wholegrain products, along with fresh meat and fish, became instantly preferable to highly processed convenience foods laden with chemical additives and preservatives.

Comfort Eating

As an antidote to feeling emotionally low, many overweight people "comfort eat." In other words they seek an endorphin rush from their food to counter feelings of depression. This became a thing of the past for me the moment I began to eat naturally, for two reasons:

Firstly, when eating naturally and focussing on taste I began to release the endorphins in my brain, not only more quickly, but also more consistently, getting a high from my food whenever I ate throughout the day, which kept me more balanced emotionally and eliminated any need to "comfort eat."

Secondly (and I believe more importantly), eating naturally involves the continual monitoring of both your TRUE level of hunger and the amount of pleasure you get from your food. As I have already said, the process of evaluation is a function of the rational mind, and when this part of the brain is activated it is easy to eat only for the right reasons; i.e. when you are feeling GENUINELY hungry, rather than emotionally low.

Comfort eating and bingeing are related, and you will find that both are eliminated when you follow the guidelines in this book.

It is worth noting that none of the naturally slim people I studied when writing this book had any desire whatsoever to comfort eat. In fact they tended to eat LESS rather than more whenever they were beset by emotional problems.

Longevity

What does eating according to the principles outlined in this book have to do with longevity?

Once you begin eating naturally your

calorie intake will reduce substantially. There have been countless laboratory experiments conducted on animals involving prolonged calorie restriction and its effects on health and longevity. To my knowledge the results have shown, without exception, that reducing calorific intake diminishes the incidence of heart disease, cancers and many other health problems – AND lengthens life considerably.

Proving conclusively that long-term calorie restriction is equally beneficial to humans is difficult because we live longer lives than laboratory animals and don't live in cages where our behaviour can be accurately monitored. However, it seems logical to me to assume that we are not much different to animals in this respect. Why should we be?

The good news is that now you have the key to permanent slimness you will certainly eat less, become slimmer, and enjoy a better quality of life. And that might make you *want* to live longer!

The Key To Permanent Slimness

What are the causes of the obesity epidemic?

The traditional line on this is the often-repeated mantra that people are eating too much fat, sugar and fast foods, and are leading sedentary lives, stuck in front of their TVs or computers. But this is not an accurate analysis of the problem. It would be possible to lead a sedentary life and stay slim if you didn't eat much, no matter how unhealthy your diet.

In my opinion, to get to the real reason why the western world is suffering from an obesity epidemic, you have to look at the key to permanent slimness, and reverse it – i.e. people do not appreciate their food enough.

The advancement in food production techniques during the last fifty years has made food much cheaper, quicker to prepare, and always available. Any time you feel hungry you can open the fridge, take out a ready-made meal, pop it in the microwave and hey presto! Dinner is served. It certainly wasn't like that years ago when people were slimmer.

The Key To Permanent Slimness

Food is no different to any other commodity – it becomes less valuable as its availability increases. We no longer take time to enjoy our food (the pre-requisite for stimulating our endorphins). Nowadays people often eat in front of the TV (modern houses are often built without dining rooms) or grab something quick and easy to prepare, which they can shovel in fast to kill off their feelings of hunger. And as we know, this invariably leads people to eat more than they need.

The French have baffled dieticians for years. They have suffered less from obesity than the rest of the western world, despite enjoying a diet of rich food. In looking at why this might be it is interesting to note that a two-hour break for lunch was until recently the norm in France. For a long time children of five years of age have been taught gastronomy in schools. Family meals around a table are still commonplace. What this tells us is that in general the appreciation of food has remained a part of French culture. Could this be why they

The Key To Permanent Slimness

have slimmer waistlines?

However, in recent years people in Paris and other metropolitan areas have begun to abandon long lunch breaks, and to accommodate this change in lifestyle, sales of fast food have increased. As you might have guessed, along with this change in eating habits has come a rise in obesity.

So it seems to me that the less you appreciate your food the more you eat and the fatter you become. Which is of course the complete opposite of the key to permanent slimness.

Now let's be brutally honest.

This book has shown you that you are no different genetically to the naturally slim, and so can become one of them. It has also shown you that dieting is *destructive* to long-term weight loss, and that exercise is inefficient as a means of curing obesity and almost impossible to stick to, especially if you are overweight. (If

The Key To Permanent Slimness

you haven't grasped these points yet, it is important that you do, and so you should read this book again).

What this means is that unless you are genuinely iron-willed, and are happy with the idea of imposing a strict dietary discipline upon your life (for the next ten, twenty, forty years, or however long you expect to live) there is NO ALTERNATIVE to the key to permanent slimness. But you will already know this because if you have bought this book you will have tried and failed to lose weight many times by using the traditional so called 'cures'.

However, many people are *unconsciously comfortable* with being continuously on a diet, despite always failing to become and stay slim, and deep down the idea of trying something new that will put an end to ALL dieting may be difficult for them to contemplate. For these people becoming slim and staying slim poses more of a problem than does being overweight. Dieting is their hobby. They love to talk about the latest one they are on, swapping notes with

The Key To Permanent Slimness

their friends. So be it. But if dieting is your pastime you would be better off <u>not</u> trying the key to permanent slimness, because it *really* does work and you will lose your hobby!

If you *genuinely* want to be slim for the rest of your life, make a deal with yourself now to try the methods outlined in this book - for just one week. Once you have experienced it there will be no going back. I have given you the key to permanent slimness. The power is in your hands. Use it or lose it. The decision is yours.

If you have a moment, please go to my website: www.permanentslimness.com and send me your feedback on this book. It would be much appreciated.

Thank you.